THERE'S A SNAKE ON MY HEAD!

Strategies for Alleviating Fear and Anxiety in Healthcare

For Patients, Families AND Healthcare Teams

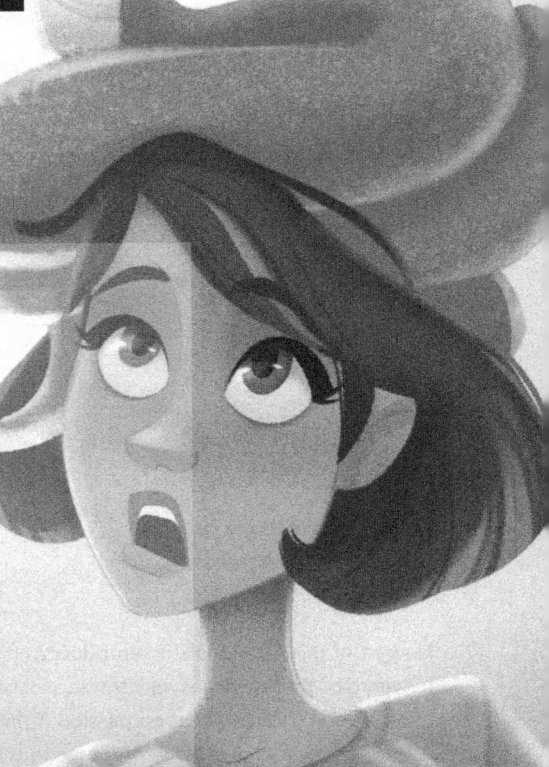

MINDY G. SPIGEL, RN, MSN, CPXP

There's a Snake on My Head!
Copyright © 2022 Mindy G. Spigel
All rights reserved.

No part of this book shall be reproduced, stored in a retrieval system, or transmitted by any means; electronic, mechanical, photocopying, recording or otherwise, without written permission from the publisher, except for providing a direct quote and providing reference to this book.

For quantity discounts, visit MindySpigel.com

ISBN: 979-8-8464-5077-6

Cover illustration: Kateryna Cherniavska • Instagram.com/kateryna.cherniavska
Production assistance: Audrey Peterson
Editing: Lydia Ramsey • LydiaRamsey.com
Cover design, interior layout, self-publishing direction: BookableMedia.com

THERE'S A SNAKE ON MY HEAD!

Strategies for Alleviating Fear and Anxiety in Healthcare

(For Patients, Families AND Healthcare Teams)

MINDY G. SPIGEL, RN, MSN, CPXP

I am dedicating this book in memory of my parents Jeanne and Marshall Gootson, who always believed in me and encouraged me to be all that I could be and to make a difference in the world. My mother always told me to do what I love and to put a lot of love into everything I do. I miss them and I feel their spirit and memory guiding me each day. They were so proud of me for becoming a nurse, and I know they would be proud of this book.

I am also dedicating this book to all the compassionate, caring, dedicated and selfless healthcare team members who do amazing things every day for patients and families. You are true heroes. I hope you find joy and fulfillment in your work, knowing that you make a difference.

Praise for *There's a Snake on My Head!*

"Mindy Spigel's work is a brilliant reminder to all healthcare providers that the work we do on a daily basis can possibly be the day that forever marks the life of the patient in our care. Our routine procedures, IV starts, delivery of a diagnosis, surgery performed, or even admitting process can be traumatizing and life changing for some patients. Patients enter a world so unfamiliar to them, though so comfortable for us—yet we have a tendency to lose sight of that. Mindy's empathetic view of the patient experience through the eyes of both patient and family is a must- read for all who are privileged enough to deliver care. It is with great hope that those who read *There's a Snake on My Head!* will never see a patient the same way again. Bravo, Mindy Spigel!"

Colleen Sweeney, RN, BS, CSP
Founder/Owner of Sweeney Healthcare Enterprises

"I have had the privilege to hear Mindy speak on the topic of patient and family fears on many occasions and have seen her inspire large groups of front-line nurses, physicians, support staff and their leaders to take the care experience to the next level. She has a unique gift of igniting compassion and empathy through a deep understanding of human behavior.

I am thrilled that she has put her expertise as a public speaker into a book so that many more can tap into this incredible passion that she has for not only the patient experience, but also the caregiver experience. It is refreshing to read a book that not only inspires the care team to identify and address patient fears, but also helps caregivers acknowledge their own fears and understand how this impacts the patients, with actionable takeaways on how to address it.

This book is an inspiring read, filled with stories and real-life examples. It is as authentic as Mindy Spigel herself and a must-read!"

Annamari Dietrichson, MHA
Division Vice President - HCA Healthcare Continental Division

"There is never a better view than from on the field vs from the bleachers! Mindy Spigel's many years as a RN, then at the bedside as a patient experience leader, educator, and trainer in many hospitals working with countless patients, their families, associates, and physicians are captured beautifully in this book. Brief and brilliant, this work provides so many "gold nuggets" on how to make the patient experience special.

The practical advice and real-life stories will help the reader easily translate these pearls of wisdom to executable actions. The winners ... your patients, their families, associates, physicians, and the honorable tradition of compassionate healthcare.

Thank you, Mindy, for sharing your experiences and wisdom. It would have been a lost opportunity to keep it to yourself for the many who can now operationalize your sage advice!"

Chris Karam, FACHE
SVP, CHRISTUS Health Louisiana - Southeast Texas

"I have had the pleasure of knowing Mindy Spigel since 2007. Her compassion and skill as a nurse is matched by her compassion for understanding the healthcare experience from the patient's point of view. Mindy's countless firsthand experiences in providing direct patient care coupled with her years of research and practice as a patient experience leader gives her a well-rounded perspective in understanding what it takes to create a truly excellent patient experience.

The stories told and lessons taught in *There's a Snake on My Head!* combine best practices with real-world practical applications to provide an easy read, but one that is full of important reminders for every healthcare professional. In an era where technology is dominating our world and all too often gets in between the caregiver and the patient, it is the simple techniques in communication and making a connection with each patient that Mindy teaches that can help every caregiver stay connected to their calling to serve others in the noble career field of healthcare."

Jeff Bourgeois, MHA, FACHE
Healthcare Executive

PRAISE FOR THERE'S A SNAKE ON MY HEAD!

"*There's a Snake on My Head!* is an important read for anyone working with and caring for patients and families. Ms. Spigel's 40+ years in healthcare lend legitimacy to her voice not always found in these types of teachings. We all create the patient and family experience, and Ms. Spigel teaches us practical, compassionate, real-world ways we can positively influence that experience. This book is effortlessly accessible and relevant, a must-read for leaders as well as practitioners in healthcare."

Trisha Montague, RN

"Mindy Spigel is a dynamic, caring nurse leader who is passionate about making a difference with nurses, physicians and patients every day. Being able to bring stories from her 40-year career to share with the audience is an incredible learning experience. Patients have fears when they come to the hospital. Being able to discuss their fears and have a listening ear can alleviate stress for the patient and their families. The caregiver then feels they have made a difference as well. The book is amazing and insightful. She is a wonderful speaker! Enjoy!"

Susan E. Osborne, RN, MSN, MBA, CPXP
Osborne Consulting

"Mindy Spigel is a talented speaker with exceptional knowledge on patient care. Mindy has the ability to convey complicated information in an easy to understand manner. Her teambuilding sessions and workshops on enhancing communication skills have been of great value to school nurses across the San Antonio area. I am excited Mindy will continue to share her knowledge through the release of her new book."

Mandy Tyler, M.Ed., RD, CSSD, LD

My Gift to You

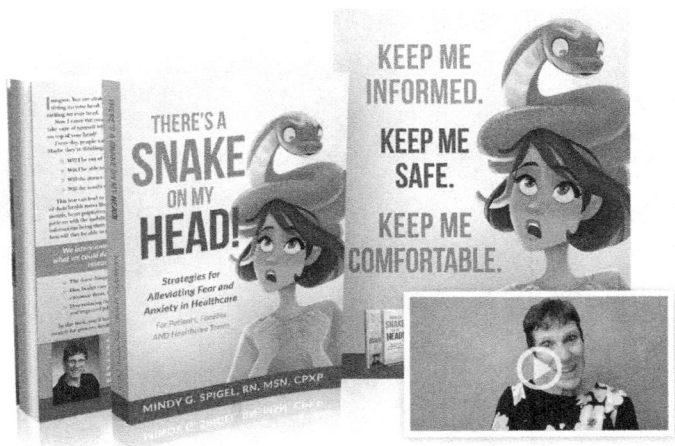

As a thank you for reading my book, I'd like to give you access to the companion training video and poster for *There's a Snake on My Head!*

In the video you'll learn:

- » Simple techniques to help put patients and families at ease without adding time to your day.
- » How they could feel more satisfied with the care they are already receiving.
- » Why they cannot hear what we are telling them, which may affect their compliance.
- » What can impact the effectiveness and job satisfaction of the healthcare team and how to resolve it.

Use the poster as a gentle reminder of what patients, families and healthcare teams need on a daily basis.

Visit **MindySpigel.com/gift**

Preface

When I retired after almost 43 years as a nurse, I was encouraged by colleagues, family and friends to write a book about what I have learned and have taught over the years. I am passionate about creating an exceptional experience for patients, families, and for clinicians whose jobs are so important and so challenging. This book is a compilation of stories and lessons.

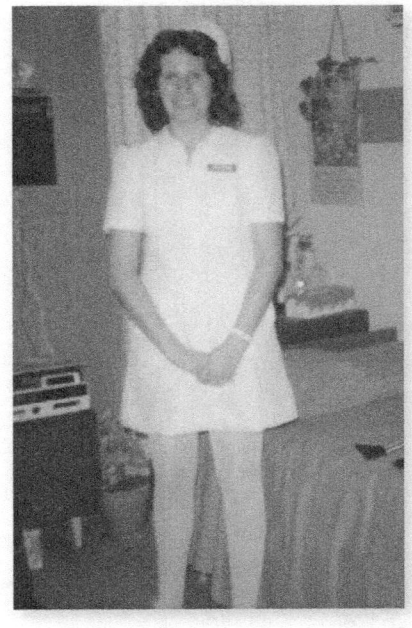

My journey really began as a young nurse, 21 or 22 years old. My first job was on a general pediatric unit of a large general hospital in the late 1970s. At that time, hospitals were not very patient and family focused. I was frustrated that parents were considered visitors and had visiting hours. I thought, "Who is really the visitor in that child's life? Their family or me?" We were offering the children an adult menu from which to order meals. Not many children eat shrimp creole. The walls were not child friendly.

One night after our shift, I was sitting in the café with colleagues, and we made a list of things we thought would make our unit better for children and families. The next morning, I took the list to our director, and, in frustration, she announced that I would need to talk to the chief nurse if I wanted to make any of these changes. Young, naïve and not realizing that nurses did not go to administration with their concerns in the late 70s, I merely replied, "Oh! Could I?"

I got that meeting, shared my concerns, and slowly things began to change. That was probably, unconsciously, a defining moment in my career. I have devoted the rest of my career striving to improve the patient experience while advocating for the creation of a culture of engagement and ownership among the clinicians and staff. Although this experience happened long before I understood fear in healthcare, I now look back and realize this was the beginning of the road to a career of alleviating fear and anxiety.

Acknowledgments

I would like to thank all the thought leaders that have influenced me. Much of what I am sharing in this book I have learned from others. Some of whom I can name, many of whom, I cannot. Their teachings have been incorporated into my life and my thinking. If I am sharing some of your story or your ideas and do not give you credit, please know it is unintentional, and I am so very grateful to you.

I would like to start with Patty Toney, who was CHRISTUS Santa Rosa Chief Nurse Executive. Besides being my mentor and friend, Patty started me on this journey. One day, she asked me to create a class on empathy. I remember wondering how in the world one would teach empathy.

Shortly later, I met Colleen Sweeney at a conference. She is an inspirational presenter and helped me on my path to understanding that patients are afraid and that empathy can impact their fear. Colleen Sweeney has been a mentor to me, and I am forever grateful to her for her kindness and generosity.

I have also been greatly influenced by Christina Dempsey, the Chief Nurse Emeritus at Press Ganey and author of *Antidote to Suffering*. I have heard her speak many times and always leave inspired. I am certain her teachings are reflected in this book.

Joe Tye, thank you for pushing me to write this book and for believing in me. Joe gave me the title for the book and pre-ordered it before the first word was even typed. I met Joe at a conference where he gave me his book, *The Florence Prescription*, which provided structure and meaning to many ideas I had about the importance of culture and creating an organizational culture of ownership and positivity. Lastly, Joe contributed a personal story for this book. Many thanks, Joe!

I must acknowledge my research team who interviewed patients and families and who contributed to the lessons I will be sharing in the book. Yesenia Ceja, BSN, RN, CPN, Amanda C. Alvarez, MSN, RN,

Ann Gonzalez, BSN, RN, CPEN and Johnny Ray Campos, RN, spent untold hours interviewing families about their fears and how we can alleviate those fears. I hope, through this book, your hard work will impact many, many patients and families beyond your own practices.

Thank you to Mary Malone. I first heard Mary speak at a conference about "Words That WOW!" Her presentation has been a part of what I teach and what I believe about words. When I started writing this book, I reached out to Mary for permission to use her story. She openly and generously offered to share anything I needed. It is people like Mary who are so committed to creating an exceptional experience for patients and families that are truly an inspiration for me.

I must thank my husband, Barry, for not only allowing me to write about him in this book, but also for being my coach, cheerleader, business manager, and best friend. Without Barry, this book would never have been completed and published.

Thank you to the team that helped me get this book into your hands. Thank you to Lisa Peterson for coordinating the publishing efforts, and Michael Meister who assisted with production and technology. Thank you to Lydia Ramsey, my editor and to Kateryna Cherniavska who illustrated the cover. You are all so talented, so patient and so very much appreciated.

Lastly, I thank and appreciate each of you, who care enough about the experience in healthcare, to pick up this book and read it. You are making a difference!

Contents

Preface xiii

Acknowledgments xv

Part 1 1

    There's a Snake on My Head! 3

    My Snake 5

    Patients and Families are Afraid 7

    Fear Relieving Strategy #1: Build a Relationship 17

    Fear Relieving Strategy #2: Choose Your Words Carefully ... 23

    Fear Relieving Strategy #3: Manage that First Impression ... 29

    Fear Relieving Strategy #4: It Takes a Team 33

    Fear Relieving Strategy #5: Technology and
    the Relationship 39

    Fear Relieving Strategy #6: Considering Different Generations
    have Different Expectations 43

Part 2 49

    Healthcare Team Members are People Too! 51

    Other Scary Times 53

    Words Matter: Their Impact on the Team 61

Final Thoughts 65

Postscript: Another Snake 67

Stories and Experiences 69

About the Author...77

Thank You! 79

What's Next?..81

Download Your Gift 83

Part 1

Part 2

There's a Snake on My Head!

Imagine. You are afraid of snakes. Terrified of snakes. Now imagine... there is a snake sitting on your head. Moving around on your head. Maybe even a rattlesnake, rattling on your head.

Now I enter your hospital room and begin to tell you important things you need to know in order to take care of yourself when you return home. How much are you going to hear when you have that snake on top of your head? I would guess not much! I first heard this story at a conference presented by Colleen Sweeney. It had an enormous impact on me and influenced my classes and workshops.

Every day, people walk into healthcare with a snake on their head. They are afraid. We do not know what frightens or worries them. It might be: Will I be out of here in time to pick up my kids? Will I be able to afford this visit? Will the clinicians be patient and kind and explain things to me? Or perhaps: Will the results of this test change my life forever? They are afraid. When they are afraid, they cannot hear all the critical things we are telling them.

Pull out your cell phone. Look at a person on your cell phone who means the world to you. Now imagine. You are traveling in a foreign country where people speak a foreign language. Suddenly, your cell phone friend becomes critically ill and ends up in a hospital in that strange country. How are you feeling right now? What are your fears? Worries? Concerns?

Every day, people come to our hospitals. To them, it is a foreign country. We speak a foreign language. We have foreign procedures. They are scared. They all have fears and concerns like you had when you thought about your loved one in that foreign country.

In this book, we will explore my journey and my research on patient and family fears. We will examine what they are telling us they need from healthcare professionals when they are afraid. I also realized that there are times when the healthcare team is afraid and needs to have their fears and anxiety addressed so that they can think clearly and be their best professional selves. We will then explore together key strategies that help minimize fear and anxiety in patients, families, and at times, members of the healthcare team.

My Snake

October 2014, my husband Barry was diagnosed with stage 3 colon cancer. Although I had been a nurse for almost 40 years, I honestly felt like he was the only person who EVER had stage 3 colon cancer. As a nurse in one of my own hospitals, I remember thinking, "I know there are other patients, but this is BARRY, and he has COLON CANCER!" I am certain that nearly everyone feels the same way—that their loved one is the sickest and most important person in the hospital.

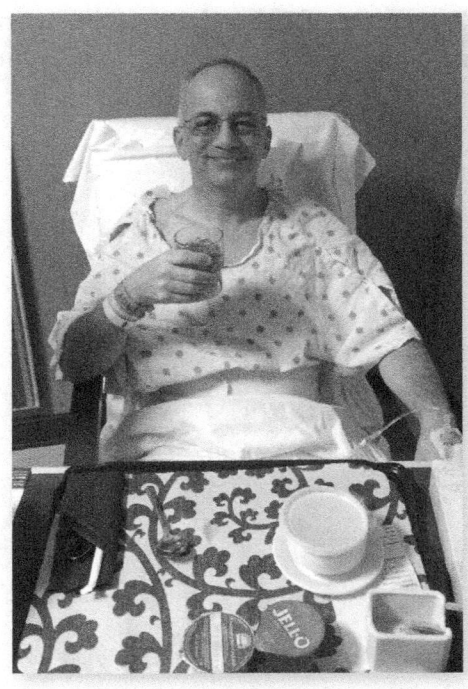

My husband was having abdominal discomfort and changes in his bowel movements. He went through months of testing for food allergies only to learn he was sensitive to fructose, something he rarely ate. The gastroenterologist suggested a colonoscopy since it had been 6 years since his last one. I could tell by the way he explained what he found during the procedure that there was more to the story. I called my primary care doctor whom I also worked with. He asked me to come to his office. It was then that he told me Barry had cancer and would need to see a colorectal surgeon. I did not hear anything else he said after that word—CANCER. That's when the snake appeared.

My husband had surgery with a fine surgeon. My primary care doctor texted me while I was waiting for Barry to come out of surgery wanting to know the results. I promised I would let him know as soon as I knew. The surgeon came out and spoke to me and my son, who was in medical school at the time. When the doctor left, I looked at my son and asked what I should text to my primary care doctor. I truly had not heard a single word the surgeon said. That snake was present.

That was just the beginning. I quickly realized I did not hear anything anyone said to me. So, I kept a notebook with important information. I would look back at my notes and declare, "They never told me that! I never heard that!" It was in my own handwriting. I listened, but I never HEARD it. I was a nurse. The hospital was not a foreign place or a foreign language for me. That snake was so real!

Patients and Families are Afraid

I first became interested in patients fears when I heard Colleen Sweeney, RN, BS speak about her work around patients' fears. One day, Sweeney was walking through her hospital when she saw a woman who seemed distraught. She asked the woman if she could help her. The woman replied that she was fine. She was at the hospital for a simple test but realized when she walked in that the last time she had been in that hospital, her mother had died there. It was not the hospital's fault she had died, but all those feelings had come back to her as she entered. Colleen realized at that moment that people are afraid; and we do not always know what they are afraid of or worried about. This moment caused Sweeney to spend three and a half years interviewing people both

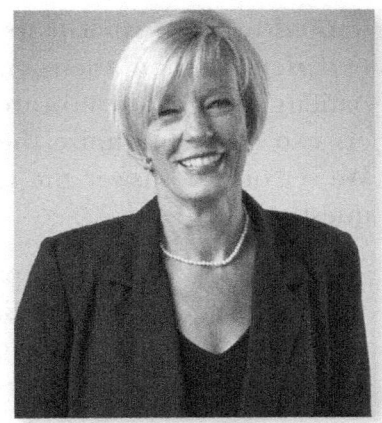

in the hospital and in the community to learn about their fears in healthcare. She found out that 96% of people are afraid. She coined the term, clinicaphobia, fear of healthcare. Sweeney is the person who introduced me to the snake analogy and has allowed me to use it in my classes and this book.

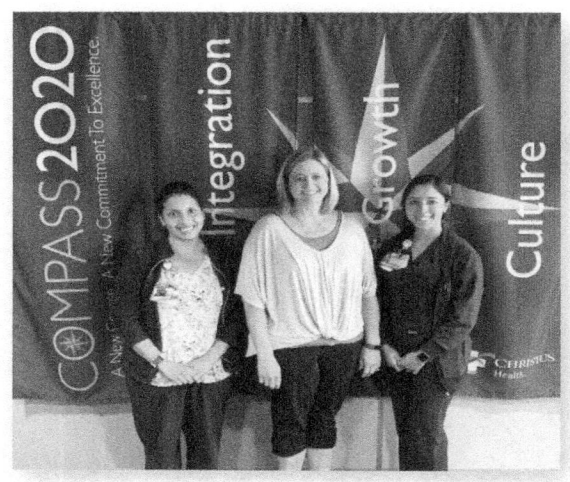

In 2018, I had the privilege of completing a research study with the help of four bilingual, pediatric nurses. This research project was generously supported by a grant from the Beryl Institute to enhance the body of knowledge about the patient experience and by CHRISTUS Children's Hospital of San Antonio. As we were expanding on Sweeney's work, we were fortunate to have her on our research team as a subject matter expert.

Acknowledging that people come into healthcare afraid and that fear can impact their ability to hear and comprehend information, we wanted to learn what fears parents experience when their child is a patient and what healthcare providers can do to minimize their fears. We set out to answer the following questions:

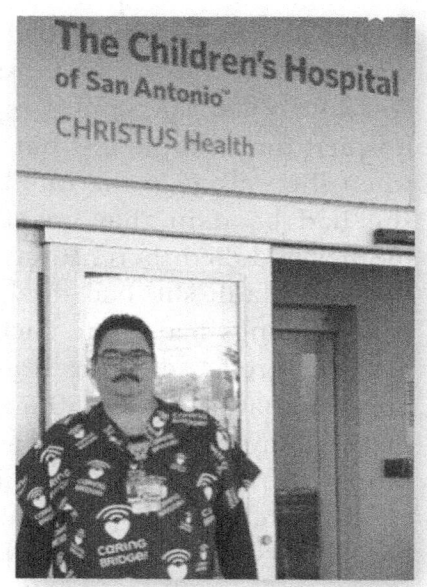

» How do the fears of parents in the healthcare setting compare to the fears of adult patients?

- » Is there a difference in parents' responses based on the setting?
- » What difference does the age of the child make?
- » What influence does primary language have on parental fears?
- » What is the most important thing we can do to decrease families' fears and concerns?

These nurses interviewed 219 families in four different settings: Emergency Department (47 families), Inpatient (87 families), Outpatient (30 families) and Perioperative Department (55 families).

They asked the parents: What were your fears or worries when you brought your child to the hospital? Of those fears, which was the most important? What is the most significant thing we can do to help alleviate your fear? The parents' responses were recorded, and themes were identified.

For our first question, how do the fears of parents in the healthcare setting compare to fears of adult patients? Sweeney found that the number one fear adults experienced was infection. For the parents, this was the third greatest fear. For the full database, the top fear was diagnosis and prognosis (50%), followed by communication issues and then infection. Interestingly, sixty percent of parents reported more than one fear.

The sample Colleen Sweeney used was not all current patients, some were adults in the community, which may have contributed to why Diagnosis and Prognosis (Will my child be ok?) was first for the parents and not the adult sample. Remember, too, this study was done in 2018 before COVID-19. The results could be different today.

Adult Fears (Colleen Sweeney)	Parental Fears (Children's Hospital of San Antonio)
Infection	Diagnosis and Prognosis (D & P)
Incompetence	Communication Issues
Death	Infection
Cost	Incompetence
Mix ups	Cost
Needles	Death
Rude Staff	Safety
Germs	Rude Staff
Prognosis and Diagnosis	Needles
Communication Issues	
Loneliness	

Fears based on location in the hospital

Across the board, in all 4 settings, we learned that all parents were afraid. The number one fear was Diagnosis and Prognosis (D & P), "Will my child be okay?" The second biggest fear was Communication, followed by Infection. Those in the surgical setting were most concerned about diagnosis and prognosis (79.4%) followed closely by infection (26.1%). This was similar for the outpatient setting.

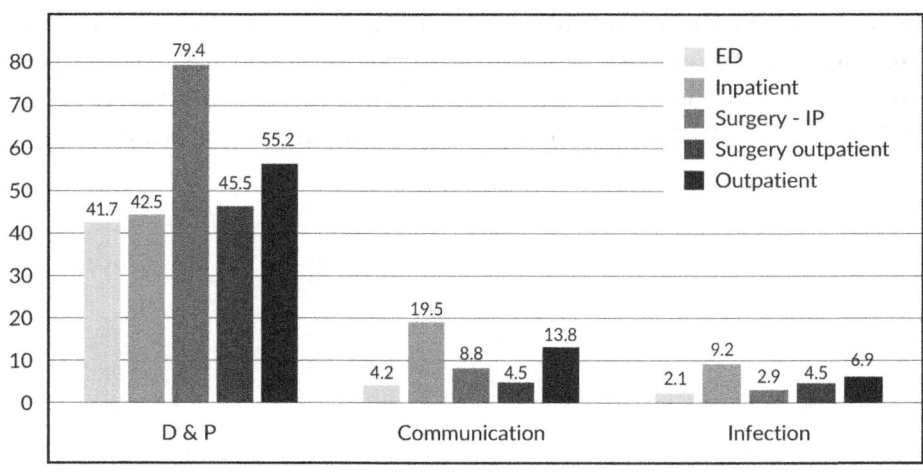

Fears based on age of patient

Although the study was done with a convenience sample of readily accessible parents, the age distribution was a good representation of the population. The interviews conducted with the parents demonstrated that there was not a statistically significant difference in the fears of the parents based on the age of the child.

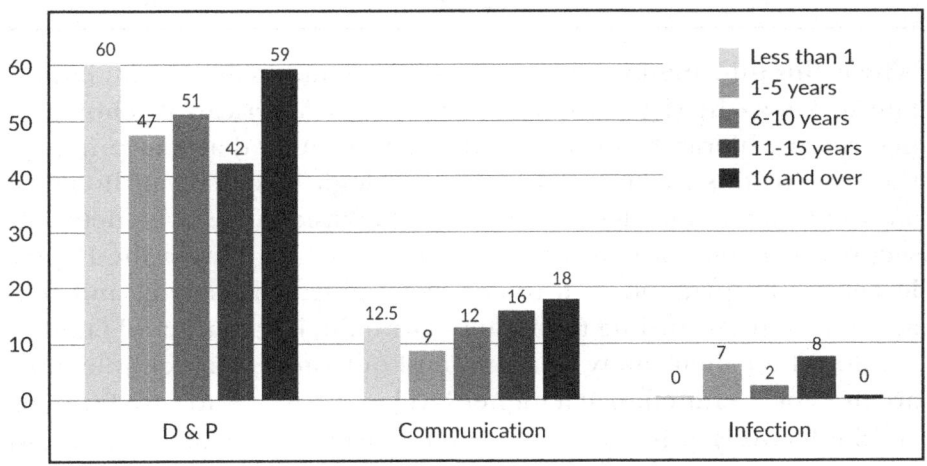

Age	Sample size
Less than 1 year	40
1-5 years	74
6 – 10 years	44
11- 15 years	43
16 +	17

As you might expect, communication was even more important with the parents who were Spanish speaking. There were 183 English-speaking parents (82%) and 36 Spanish-speaking parents (18%) in this study. As expected, Spanish speakers were more concerned about communication than their English-speaking counterparts. When looking at the first 3 fears combined, 76.5% of Spanish speakers were concerned about communication and 37.3% of English speakers were concerned about communication.

	English	Spanish
Communication as 1st fear	10.3%	22.9%
Communication as 2nd fear	13.5%	28.6%
Communication as 3rd fear	13.5%	25.0%
Total	**37.3%**	**76.5%**

Why is this information, that patients and families are afraid, important to know? In 1943, Abraham Maslow, an American Psychologist, described a hierarchy of human needs represented as a pyramid. At the base of this pyramid are the physiologic needs of all humans: air, food, water, and sleep. Just above the basic needs are safety and security. If people are afraid, they are unable to achieve the higher levels on the pyramid of love and belonging, self-esteem, and self-actualization. According to Maslow's pyramid, if patients and families are afraid for their safety, comfort, and outcomes, for example, they are not able to function at a higher level to learn how to care for their child effectively at home. This model explains why when I was afraid

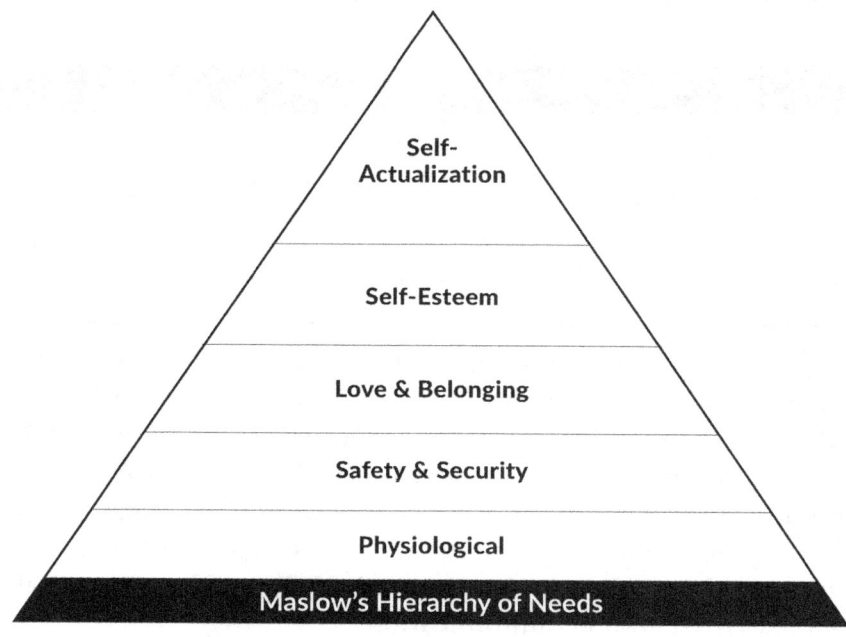

PATIENTS AND FAMILIES ARE AFRAID

that my husband could die from his colon cancer or surgery, I did not remember information that was shared with me by the healthcare team.

The most powerful part of the study, I believe, has to do with the last question, "What is the most important thing we can do to alleviate your fear?" Across the board, in all settings, we heard:

- » Keep me informed.
- » Keep me safe.
- » Keep me comfortable.

When you think about your cell phone person in a hospital, is that not what you want for them?

As I learned that these were the most important things to families, I suddenly realized that was why the well-established best practices like how we introduce ourselves, frequent rounding on patients and handoffs at the bedside involving the patient and family, and use of the communication board in the patient's room are so important. These best practices support keeping people safe and comfortable while keeping them informed.

A friend of mine recently shared a letter she wrote to a hospital following gallbladder surgery. I highlighted a few key words.

> *I was experiencing excruciating abdominal pain. After I fainted from the pain, my husband called 911. The paramedics informed me that I would be taken to our local hospital. My reaction was "Oh no! It is way too small." I was **frightened** but trusted the paramedics.*
>
> *When I arrived at the Emergency Room, I had a wonderful experience. After my situation was diagnosed, I was **informed** that my gallbladder had to be removed. My surgeon stopped by my room to **introduce himself and put my mind at ease** with his **wonderful bedside manner** and tremendous **knowledge**.*

My friend was afraid. Information and compassion put her at ease.

During my first review of the results with the research team, they shared some interesting stories.

One nurse on the research team shared that during the study, her child became ill. She took her child to the Emergency Department of her hospital. She reported that being a parent of a child in the hospital changed her perspective. On her way to the hospital, she was afraid and wondered, "Did I do the right thing bringing her in with a stomachache?" When her daughter was diagnosed with appendicitis, she worried, "Did I wait too long?" She realized that parents are fearful of being judged for not being a good parent.

Another researcher said that the study made her a better nurse. She realized how overwhelming it is for families to have a loved one in the hospital. She realized how important bedside handoffs and involving the patient and family in the care planning were. She also noted that team rounding was critically important since it is frightening for patients if they are receiving different information from different care team members. It is important that the information shared is consistent and understood. Lastly, she noted that it is important to update the patient and family on their progress and the plan of care more often than every 12 hours.

Keep me informed.
Keep me safe.
Keep me comfortable.

When I was a patient in the hospital, the communication board in the room was a dynamic tool. I was only in the inpatient room for about 15 hours. The plan was changed and updated at least three times. I knew exactly what I needed to do to be able to go home, and I knew how I was progressing on the checklist. It was reassuring.

Lastly, a researcher noted that we cannot guess what patients and families are worried about. We must ask them. It should be a routine part of every clinician's care to assess their worries and fears so we may address them. It is also important to assess the most important action we can take to address their fear from their perspective. Sweeney advises that we not ask a person what their fears are, as fear is something people hold close. Rather, ask, "What is your greatest concern or worry that I might help you with today?" In response, they will readily share their fear.

When you see people who are angry, it is important to remember that under that anger is often fear. Fear displays itself as anger. Our tendency as humans confronted by someone who is angry is to push back or flee. People who are afraid do not want us to do either of those things. Take a moment to ask them about their biggest worry or concern at that moment and what you might do to help them. It may alleviate their fear and anxiety and diminish their anger.

Based on the learnings from the research study, let's explore some strategies that help people feel informed, safe and comfortable, thereby easing their fear and anxiety.

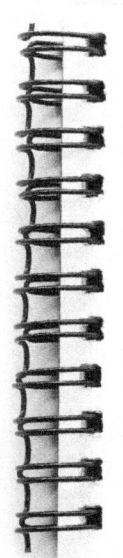

Action Steps

- » *Recognize that patients and families in all healthcare settings are afraid or worried.*
- » *Keep patients and families informed, safe, and comfortable.*
- » *Ask patients and families, "What are your greatest worries or concerns?"*
- » *Remember that people who are angry are often afraid, so ask them what they are worried or stressed about.*

Fear Relieving Strategy #1:
Build a Relationship

I will always remember the story I was told about a nurse who was off for several days. Upon her return, she was given "the difficult patient" because she was fresh. This patient was angry and demanding and pushed the call button frequently. The nurse prioritized spending some time with him. She pulled up a chair and sat down to talk to him for a few minutes. She learned that he was 30 years old and was afraid he was dying of cancer. The most amazing thing was that after a few minutes of conversation, he was no longer difficult with her. They had a relationship. She knew his biggest fear. He knew she cared.

Patients want you to know them as a person. When we take a moment to know that person, not as the patient in room 10, but as a former CEO, a successful tennis player, a grandmother or the owner of a beautiful cat, it makes a difference. When we know them as a person, they feel valued, cared about and important. When I was having surgery at one of my hospitals, everyone knew me and treated me as a special friend. That is exactly the experience that everyone wants. How do we create that experience in the middle of our busyness?

First, be sure to introduce yourself in a way that puts patients and families at ease. Not just your name, include your role in words that express how passionate you are about taking great care of them. Smile while introducing yourself. Even if you are wearing a mask, a smile shows in your eyes and changes the tone of your voice. The next time you answer the phone or you see someone wearing a mask, ask yourself if you think that person is smiling. You can tell.

If you have a scribe or student with you, be sure to introduce them as well. People are wondering who is listening to their story and health concerns. I was having an echocardiogram done one day. I believe the cardiologist expected to see something interesting. In the middle of the procedure, the door opened and the cardiologist plus a parade of students or residents came in. They were all fixated on the screen, not even acknowledging that I was on the table. After I said something, the student at the end of the line looked at me, introduced themself and said hello. Can you imagine how I felt? I was being seen as an object on a screen rather than as me the person.

> *When we listen with the intent to understand, rather than the intent to reply, we begin true communication and relationship building.*
>
> *Opportunities to then speak openly and to be understood come much more naturally and easily.*
>
> Stephen R. Covey
> The 7 Habits of Highly Effective People: Powerful Lessons in Personal Change

Make eye contact while introducing yourself. It builds a connection. Someone once said, "When your eyes connect, your hearts connect." I believe that. Do not let your paper or computer distract you. Notice the family members in the room as well. They are a part of the team. A moment of eye contact begins to build trust.

Sit down if possible. When you are at eye level, you connect. People often say that when one person is standing and the other is sitting, it feels like they are talking AT you. When they sit down, it feels like they are talking WITH you. Try it. Ask your colleague to talk to you while you are sitting and they are standing. Then ask them to repeat it while both of you are sitting. Powerful.

FEAR RELIEVING STRATEGY #1: BUILD A RELATIONSHIP

My husband went for a follow up visit with a physician and reported to me that the physician was standing during the visit, and he was sitting. After a short time, my husband was so uncomfortable, that he stood up to be at eye level with the physician.

One day, I asked a physician and a nurse in one of our Emergency Rooms to pose for a couple of photos with me to use in a presentation I was preparing for a group of physicians. I handed my cell phone to another nurse, and she quickly took these two photos. I think a picture is worth a thousand words. What do you think? Can you feel the difference? In which situation do you think I would be most likely to ask the physician a question?

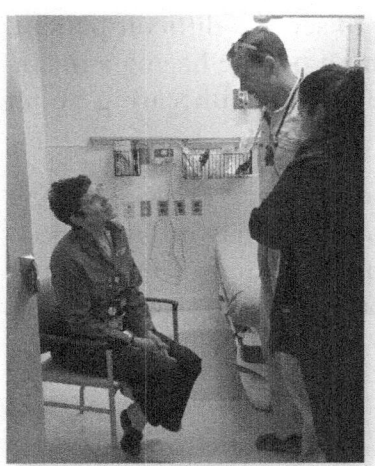
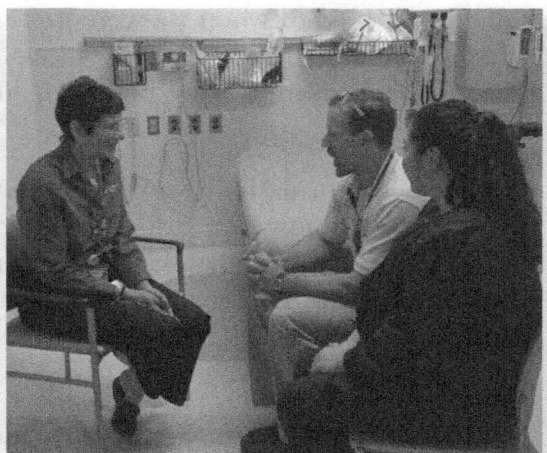

We must ask the patient what is most important to them, and we must listen to their response. Listen with the intent to understand and not the intent to reply. You may learn about their greatest fears and worries and be able to put them at ease.

Always know one thing about your patient that is not the reason for their visit or why they are in the hospital. If you know that one thing, it builds the relationship. One day, I was going to visit a patient and the nurse told me that "one thing" before my visit. This patient had done some important things in her life. When I walked in and showed an interest in wanting to learn about her and her life experience, we immediately connected.

Another day, I was offering coaching on bedside shift report and planned to follow a team of nurses. The offgoing nurse asked that I not come with them into a particular patient's room as he was "a difficult patient." I told the nurse I had confidence in him and he was the patient I wanted to meet. When we entered the room, the nurse introduced us to the patient and told us that this gentleman had a beautiful cat. On cue, the man pulled out his phone and shared a photo of his cat. The oncoming nurse asked the name of the cat and instantly there was a bond. The three of them discussed the man's care, his progress and the plan for the day. As we walked out, I asked when we were going to see the difficult patient. I had not seen a difficult patient. I saw three people having a meaningful conversation. I truly believe it all started with caring about a cat.

When meeting a patient, introduce yourself. Make eye contact. Sit down. Listen. Know one thing about them that has nothing to do with their health. It only takes a few minutes to build trust and put the patient at ease so you can get that snake off their head, and they can hear you.

And if you are a leader, remember that all of this is very important for our associates as well. They want you to know them. If they walk into your office, look up. Eye contact matters. Be on the same level as you talk with them. Listen to their worries and concerns. Know something about them that has nothing to do with their job.

For team members, this is important to your colleagues. Whether they are from your department or a department that supports you, learn something about them. Greet them when you see them. Make eye contact and listen to them. Thank them for helping you. When you acknowledge someone for helping you, they go home at the end of the day feeling more fulfilled and are more likely to help you in the future.

FEAR RELIEVING STRATEGY #1: BUILD A RELATIONSHIP

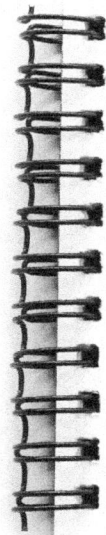

Action Steps

» *Introduce yourself.*
» *Make eye contact and smile.*
» *Sit down.*
» *Listen, truly listen.*
» *Know one thing about the patient that is not the reason for the visit.*

Fear Relieving Strategy #2:
Choose Your Words Carefully

As we begin to look at the power of words, I believe it is important to begin with ourselves. What do we say to ourselves each day? Our brain is listening and wants us to be right. I love flying on Southwest Airlines. That is my preferred airline. One day I needed to fly on another airline as Southwest did not go to my destination. I arrived at the airport and had to "pay for my bags." I knew I would need to pay for my bags, but that did not stop me from thinking, "Southwest does not charge me for my bags!" I got to the gate as they began to board. Boarding groups 1 and 2 were invited to board down the red carpet. By the time they got to my boarding group, I was invited to walk along the wall next to the red carpet since I had not paid for the privilege of the red carpet. Again, I thought, "Not on Southwest where everyone is a first-class passenger!" The flight attendant did not make the announcements the same way as the peppy Southwest flight attendants, nor did they take the drink orders in the same manner.

At that point, I realized what I was doing so I said to myself, "Stop it! Did they board the plane on time? Did they take off safely? Has the flight gone smoothly?" I realized that when I woke that morning, I had told myself, "Ugh, this will not be a Southwest experience." My brain wanted me to be right and had worked hard to find all the ways this flight was going to be different. That is when I realized the power of the words we use when talking to ourselves. How can we use this lesson of the power of words with our families?

We can use this concept in a positive way. If what patients and families want from us is to keep them informed, keep them safe and keep them comfortable, then we can use those words. "I am going to keep you safe." It already makes them feel safe and what does their brain do? It looks for everything we do to keep them safe. "I care about your comfort." Now, not only do they begin to see how we are keeping them comfortable, but they also know we care about them as well. "I am going to keep you informed about your care. I will let you know what to expect all along the way."

What happens when patients and families hear, "We are short staffed today" or "I have a lot of other patients"? AT&T ran a great series of commercials in 2019 about how okay is not okay. One commercial had to do with a patient who was going for surgery and asked the nurse if their doctor was good. Her response was "He's okay." Do you want surgery by a doctor who is "just okay"? You could see the patient's and his wife's fear increase as the nurse said those words.

Many years ago, I heard Mary Malone speak at a conference. She shared a story about a father who needed surgery.

The day before surgery, he came to the hospital with his daughter for lab work and to complete the paperwork. Every person who picked up his paperwork remarked, "Oh, your doctor is a great doctor and really nice guy too!" They went home that day feeling at ease about the upcoming surgery. They felt they had selected the right doctor and the right hospital.

The next day at the hospital, the dad was in bed and the daughter was sitting beside him when the nurse walked by the door. She noticed that the dad was still in the room. She muttered under her breath, never dreaming that the dad and daughter would hear her, "Those idiots in transport. Where are they?" The

FEAR RELIEVING STRATEGY #2: CHOOSE YOUR WORDS CAREFULLY

dad looked at his daughter and said, "They have idiots here. They know they have idiots here. I hope there are no idiots in surgery."

The words we use can have the power to put people at ease or make them afraid.

Every weekend, I go to a vegetable stand that is near my home to purchase fresh vegetables. The young man who runs the stand is in his 20s and has amazing customer service skills. He greets me each week as though his best friend has arrived and when he tells me how much I owe him, he says, "For YOU, that will be…" I do believe he gives me a discount as a frequent customer and the words "for YOU" make me feel special. If too many weeks go by that I have not gone to his vegetable stand, I feel bad. I feel like my visits matter to him.

Patients and families want to know they are special and matter to us. When we say "Let me get that for YOU," it has the same effect. They feel valued, cared for and cared about; all of which helps to remove the snake. Remember that to every patient and family member, they or their loved one is the sickest, most important person.

At almost 65 years old, I had my first real surgery. I had been a nurse for over 40 years yet the only time I had been hospitalized was for the birth of my children. I was scared. In the preoperative area, I shared my feelings with the nurse caring for me. She sat down near me, took my hand and told me that she would keep me informed about what to expect. She said she would be with me the whole way, and we would have plenty of time together before surgery. She assured me that my physician and my anesthesiologist were the best. It immediately alleviated my fears, and I felt safe. Even though I had taught this concept for years, when I was on the other side, I realized how truly powerful information is in helping people feel in control and not so frightened.

What if that nurse had said, "You should be scared," or "Your doctor is okay," or "I have other patients, you know"? Words matter. Choose yours carefully.

Be mindful about setting time expectations. When you say "I will be back in a minute" to the patient, that means 60 seconds. What does that usually mean to us? Soon. When 60 seconds pass, I can assure you that minute is much longer to someone waiting than it is to the busy clinician. You have not kept your promise. That impacts trust.

One day, I was getting my blood drawn at one of the hospitals where I worked. The technician said, "Have a seat in the lounge. I will be there in a sec." I thought to myself, no need to sit down if it is going to be a second. When I opened the door to the lounge and saw several people waiting, I realized it would not be a second so I sat down. Choose your words wisely. Always tell people it will take longer than you truly expect. That way, when you are there earlier than they expected, they will be pleasantly surprised.

It is important to keep people informed about delays. We get embarrassed about keeping people waiting, especially if they are waiting on us. It is important to that patient and family to know that we have not forgotten them. If you keep them informed about delays, they can tolerate the wait much better.

If they have been waiting on you, acknowledge the wait and apologize for the inconvenience. I have two stories that illustrate this point. My husband had to have a port placed for his chemotherapy following surgery. The hospital required that we arrive two hours before the procedure. My husband is the type of person who arrives 15 minutes early so he will not be late. You can imagine that two hours later when the nurse came in and told us that the surgeon was running an hour late, my husband was upset. He was anxious so waiting two hours was an eternity. When the surgeon arrived, he thumbed through the chart and said, "Looks like you are all set. See you in surgery." No apology. Six months later when it was time to take the port out, we asked his colorectal surgeon if he could do it for us. All because of a missed apology.

The second story is about me. I have this magical hour I made up in my head. For any doctor's appointment, I expect to be out one hour after my appointment time. One year, during my annual appointment

FEAR RELIEVING STRATEGY #2: CHOOSE YOUR WORDS CAREFULLY

with my gynecologist, 45 minutes into my magic hour, I am on the table, in a gown, vital signs taken and no further word. I begin to talk to myself about leaving. On the one hand, I have a busy day ahead, I need to get back to work, this is taking too long. And on the other hand, I tell myself, if you leave now, you will need to block out time to make another appointment and do this all over again. While I am arguing with myself, the gynecologist walks in and takes my hand, sits down and says, "Ms. Mindy, I am so sorry for keeping you waiting. My last patient needed a little extra time. I hope I have not inconvenienced you." I immediately replied, "Oh no problem!" No problem? A minute earlier, I was mentally getting dressed, preparing to leave and now, it was no problem. Why? All because she apologized and acknowledged the inconvenience. Words matter. Choose yours carefully.

> *Kind words can be short and easy to speak, but their echoes are truly endless.*
>
> Mother Teresa

One last tip, instead of asking "Do you have any questions?" ask, "What questions do you have for me?" I have had the honor of shadowing hospitalists and Emergency Room physicians, and I have noticed they almost always ask the first version of this question. As a nurse, I can tell you that patients will most often shake their head "no" when asked if they have questions. They have a snake on their head. They do not hear what you say, but they do not want to look stupid or disappoint you. When you walk out of the room, they will often look at their nurse and ask, "What did they just say?" When you say, "We have been through a lot of information, and I want to make sure I was clear. What questions do you have for me?" it infers that most people have questions. If you are seated, they are highly likely to ask you the questions that are on their mind. ***Words Matter.***

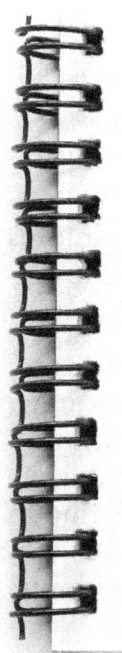

Action Steps

- » Choose your words carefully. Words have the power to put people at ease or make them afraid.
- » Be careful about the words you say to yourself. Your brain is listening and wants you to be right.
- » Use words to alleviate patient and family fears: I will keep you safe. I will keep you comfortable. I will keep you informed. Patients will notice everything you do to prove those points.
- » Emphasize "For YOU" to make patients feel special.
- » Underpromise and overdeliver when speaking about time. Apologize for any delays.
- » Ask, "What questions do you have for me?" instead of "Do you have any questions?"

Fear Relieving Strategy #3:
Manage that First Impression

At the start of the COVID-19 pandemic, my husband and I chose to be careful to minimize our risk. For eight months, we avoided stores, restaurants, and indoor gatherings. In November 2020, we took a driving trip from Texas to the East Coast to see family.

The first night we stopped at a hotel a bit uncertain and armed with wipes to sanitize our room. We were greeted by a receptionist who was behind plexiglass and wearing a mask with hand sanitizer on the counter. We got to our room where there was a seal on the door that we broke to enter. Once inside there was a list of the things that had been done to ensure our room was clean. We both exhaled as we felt safe.

The second night (same hotel chain, new city), we got to the registration desk to find no plexiglass and no face mask being worn by the receptionist. My husband commented to her. She replied that she had three masks with her. In the hallway, we met a housekeeper also without a mask. Our hotel room door did not have a seal on it. We were both extremely uncomfortable so I pulled out my wipes. Now, I bet that both rooms had been cleaned the same way, but it was our first impression that set the tone for whether we felt safe.

In the healthcare setting, what is the first impression that patients and families get when they enter? Do we help them feel safe or feel afraid? Do we warmly welcome people and put them at ease, or do we process them, leaving them feeling like we do not care?

One year, I went for my mammogram to a facility I had never been to before. When I walked in, I warmly greeted the receptionist who looked up and said, "Do you have an appointment?" When I replied that I did, she asked for my insurance card and driver's license and quickly made copies of both. When done, she returned them and directed me to a chair and said that someone would be out to get me shortly. She was efficient, but there was never a moment of warmth or caring. I was processed, not greeted. How much effort does it take to look up, make eye contact, smile, and say good morning before asking for an insurance card?

I always tell registration staff members that they are the Directors of First Impressions. They are the first people that patients and families meet when they enter your facility. People use that interaction to unconsciously make an assessment about your facility. Is this a place that genuinely cares? Remember, people want us to keep them informed, keep them safe and keep them comfortable. It begins with the first encounter. I once left a physician's practice because I did not like the way I was treated by the front office staff. They had a glass window, and when they were finished with you, they slammed it shut. They were curt on the phone. I loved the physician and the team in the back, but dreaded dealing with the front office. Think of all the time you spend with the front office staff. Often it is longer than the amount of time spent with the staff in the back.

Registration staff should always look up when people enter, even if they are on the phone, making eye contact, smiling and looking like they are happy to see them. Once in a store, I walked up to the customer service counter. Everyone was busy, nobody even looked up or

FEAR RELIEVING STRATEGY #3: MANAGE THAT FIRST IMPRESSION

acknowledged my husband and I standing at the counter. I said to my husband, "Oh, I must be invisible again. I hate being invisible." We never want scared patients and families to feel invisible. They understand if you are busy, just acknowledge that you see them and will get back to them in a moment.

Take a moment for small talk. "Beautiful day today, isn't it?" "Did you have a nice weekend?" "I love your beautiful necklace." These simple words communicate that you know there is a person in front of you and not just another number. If it is obvious that the person is not feeling well, acknowledge that you are sorry they are ill, but that they are in the right place and that the team will take great care of them. Treat them as you would treat someone who came into your home. You would always start with a nice greeting and not merely, "Who are you here to see?" Once registered, it is important to tell patients what and whom to expect next. Now that they trust you and know you care about them, they extend that trust to the next person they will meet.

> Don't walk in front of me, I may not follow. Don't walk behind me, I may not lead. Just walk beside me and be my friend.
>
> Philosopher Albert Camus

Look around your space. What is the first impression people get when they enter your department? Is there clutter and chaos? Is it warm and inviting? Does it look like you care? As you walk around your facility, make it a point to keep your eyes up and not looking at a document or a phone. When we pass people in the hallway without noticing them, it is common to feel invisible, and nobody likes to feel invisible. You may be missing a chance to be helpful. The person you are passing may be lost or confused. Make a point to notice and offer your assistance. It communicates that we care.

What do people hear when they are in your department? They are listening and hear everything that is being said. Everything they hear affects them. Do they hear:

» We are short staffed today.
» What a busy day, everyone is sick!

- » The doctor is slow.
- » I wish I was at home today.
- » That patient is so difficult.

What do you want them to hear?

When you walk a patient and family back to a room, do you have them follow you or walk beside you?

A famous saying often attributed to philosopher Albert Camus says, "Don't walk in front of me, I may not follow. Don't walk behind me, I may not lead. Just walk beside me and be my friend." Whenever possible, walk beside people. Use this as an opportunity to make small talk, to establish a connection and put them at ease.

We have all heard that you only have one chance to make a first impression. What is not clear is how long it takes to make that first impression. Depending on what you read, the number of seconds vary, but it takes only *SECONDS* to make a first impression. When you see a stranger somewhere, notice how long it takes to determine if they seem friendly, helpful, approachable. What are people's first impressions of you? What do you want them to be? First impressions matter.

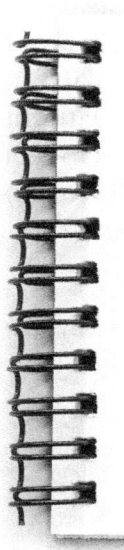

Action Steps

- » Manage your first impression carefully.
- » Always look up and greet people warmly when they approach your desk, or you pass them in the hallway.
- » Welcome people; never just process them.
- » Take a moment for small talk. Get to know them as a person.
- » Remember that people hear everything being said around them. What do you want them to hear?

Fear Relieving Strategy #4:
It Takes a Team

I mentioned earlier that after being a nurse for over 40 years and having just retired as the Director of Patient Experience, I had my first surgery at one of my hospitals in the middle of the Covid pandemic. I switched doctors for my surgery because my gynecologist did not have privileges at my hospital. She referred me to a colleague who had privileges there. I chose the hospital over my physician. Consequently, I had high expectations for the care I would receive at this hospital.

One week after my surgery, I wrote the following letter to the president and chief nurse of the hospital (names have been removed for their privacy):

> *As you know, I chose your hospital over my physician for my surgery because I knew that I would receive exceptional care. You did not disappoint. I was treated like royalty! More importantly, I can tell that the way I was treated is truly your standard of care and a cut above the norm. I experienced the WOW factor over and over again.*

The things that stand out to me are teamwork and information. I saw that in preadmission testing, again in Pre-op, meeting the OR team and on the inpatient unit. What I want your team to know is that teamwork and information truly help the patient feel safe. Let me explain:

In preadmission testing (PAT), I felt like the entire team took care of me. The handoffs were seamless. It was a well-oiled machine with large doses of compassion. I never felt rushed even though you were incredibly busy that afternoon. Everyone took time to explain exactly what was going to happen while in PAT. They made sure I totally understood how to prepare for surgery. I felt confident that they knew how to do it right when they were done.

The day of surgery, the pre-op experience could not have been better. When I walked in, a nurse I knew well greeted me and told me that she had requested to work that day so she could take care of me in recovery. It made me feel safe going into surgery knowing she would be there when I woke up! Unfortunately, I do not remember my time with her in recovery other than the transfer to the floor, but I know she took great care of me.

My pre-op nurse was amazing. There is no doubt in my mind why her patients love her. I told her it was my first surgery, and I was scared. She told me she would help me. She told me we had lots of time to get ready. She explained everything that would happen. I knew exactly what would occur and in what order even when she went to cover PACU. She listened, she comforted, she made me feel safe and cared for. She told me how much she loves her patients and how passionate she is about helping them feel at ease. It is obvious.

What a treat to have my OR nurse come to the pre op area from the OR to prepare me for that part. Once again, she repeated that she was part of a team. She told me exactly what I could expect to happen and put me at ease. Unfortunately, I do not remember the OR team, but I do want to say thank you for taking care of me. And the chaplain,

FEAR RELIEVING STRATEGY #4: IT TAKES A TEAM

what a gift to this organization. She knows exactly what to say to relieve patients' anxiety before surgery.

I was amazed that both the hospitalist and the inpatient nurse came to see me in pre-op and told me they would take care of me on the inpatient side. Unfortunately, my surgery was delayed, and I did not see the nurse who came by because it was already the night shift. I felt safe and comforted knowing she would be there when I arrived. It was a great touch. As for the hospitalist I saw that night - WOW! He did everything exactly right. As you know, I coach hospitalists. I am not sure what I could do to coach him. He even managed up the nursing team. Again, he was not there the next day, so I never saw him again, but he was reassuring at the time. The hospitalist on my second day was wonderful as well and took time to make sure that I had the help I needed at home.

The recovery room nurse took me to the floor and gave her report at the bedside so my husband Barry and I could both hear. I must admit, I do not remember much about it except that it was comforting to have that handoff.

> Alone we can do so little; together we can do so much.
>
> Helen Keller

The time on the floor with both the night nurse and the day nurse, and the two very attentive CNAs who worked with them could not have gone any better. I felt listened to, respected, cared about, and safe. Once again, everything was explained to me. I knew exactly what the plan was for each shift. The communication board was used exactly as it is intended, including the respiratory therapist who set up my incentive spirometer. The night nurse started the plan and updated it as needed. Once the day nurse came in, they did the bedside shift report exactly as it is supposed to be done. When the day nurse came to my bedside to hear report with me, I felt so much respect and caring and like the most important person in the room. When the report was done, she immediately updated the board not only with names but what needed to be accomplished for me to go home that day. Both nurses listened to me and cared about my thoughts and feelings. This compassion and respect mean so much when you are the person in the bed. I must go one step further. I totally felt that the entire team cared for every patient on the floor. If I pushed the call button, it was answered immediately. When I was in the bathroom, I was told for my safety to pull the call bell and wait for someone. When I did, a nurse was there instantly. She had no idea it was me. She was just keeping the patient in room 245 safe. When I told her my concerns, she said she would let my nurse know and very soon, my nurse was in my room AND already knew everything that had happened. That is teamwork. And teamwork is what truly helps patients feel safe and comfortable and valued.

I would be remiss if I did not mention my experience with food service, especially at breakfast. I called to order breakfast, but my diet order had not been advanced in the system yet. I mentioned it to the nurse who immediately changed the order. Here is what amazed me...the dietary team called me before I even had a chance to call them again. They did everything perfectly in terms of taking my order, delivering my order, and the food was delicious. It was exactly as I have taught over and over again. I really do not think they knew who I was. Everyone from food service to housekeeping to the nursing team never left my room without asking if I needed anything. I never felt that anything was "not my job." I have often heard complaints that trays were delivered without moving things close by or offering to assist with opening things. I did not experience that at all.

I have read about all these issues on surveys over the years, but only when you are on the receiving end do you really understand. The staff works as a team, and they appear to love what they do. Although, I knew the floor was busy while I was there, I felt like the only patient. I have read that comment many times before on your surveys.

My research conducted last year on 225 families showed that what scared patients and families want in the hospital is to be informed, safe and comfortable. Look at how many times I have used those words in my story. You are amazing, and I am so proud to have been a part of your organization. I have said countless times before that

FEAR RELIEVING STRATEGY #4: IT TAKES A TEAM

you are a beautiful hospital, but the work you do is so much more than just that. Beautiful things are happening inside the building. Never stop doing what you are doing, it is too important.

In my letter, I hope you noticed that it took every team member and every encounter to create this experience that made me feel safe and comfortable. Many of the team members managed up the next person I would be encountering. They worked together to create a seamless experience. Teamwork. So powerful at creating a sense of safety and removing the snake!

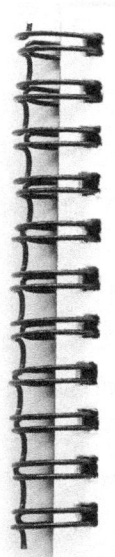

Action Steps

» Make people feel safe and comfortable.

» Take special care to include the patient and family in our handoffs.

» Manage up the other members of the team that the patient will encounter.

» Remember that every member of the team is important and every encounter matters.

» Never say "not my job" or "not my patient." All patients and families need us.

Fear Relieving Strategy #5:
Technology and the Relationship

Technology, both a great tool and a possible impediment to creating a great experience and a great connection.

I would like to start with the telephone. Often, this is the first impression a person has with your organization. What impression do they get? What impression do you want them to have? I am thinking we want them to feel connected and cared for. Calling a healthcare organization is not something we look forward to doing. People are scared, worried, and dreading the visit. How can the person on the phone begin the process of alleviating that fear?

My first tip is to stop, make eye contact with the phone and put a smile on your face when you answer. The next time you are talking to someone on the phone, ask yourself, "Are they smiling?" Smiling softens your voice quality making your voice sound warmer and more inviting. Here's a quick exercise: pretend to answer the phone without smiling. Now, say the same thing with a smile on your face. Sound different? I bet it does.

THERE'S A SNAKE ON MY HEAD!

What about eye contact with the phone? One day, I was working on the PowerPoint for a presentation I was preparing when my phone rang. I reached over to answer without looking away from the computer and said, "This is Mindy Gootson. How may I help you?" It had been over 20 years since I had been married, and yet I unconsciously answered using my maiden name. Have you ever shared your story with someone on the phone, and when you were finished, they asked you questions, all of which you had just answered? We do not multitask as well as we think. When we make eye contact with the phone, even briefly, it switches our brain focus from what we had been doing to what we are now doing.

Even with a smile and eye contact, the words we choose and our voice quality matter. This may be the 200th time today that you are scheduling an appointment for someone, but it is their first time. This call matters to the person on the other side. Find a way to connect with them. For example, "I am sorry you are not feeling well. Let me see how soon we can get you in." My birthday is March 4, 1956. I always say 3-4-5-6 when asked for a birthdate. People who are paying attention and not just processing me catch it. They comment, and we build a connection. Always end the conversation on a warm note: "I hope you have a great day" or "I hope you feel better soon." Just make it something personal.

Once you learn the name of the person on the phone (or in person), be sure to use it as often as you can. It personalizes the encounter, and it makes them feel special.

One word about putting someone on hold. Here's a pet peeve of mine: "This is _____, can you hold please?" Click. I usually look at the phone without anyone actively on the other end and reply "No, I can't hold." How much longer does it take to wait for a reply? When you return to the caller after putting them on hold, thank them for waiting. Remember that their time is important as well.

One of the advancements of 2020 was certainly televisits. They are great tools for bringing healthcare to people who may not be able to travel. During the pandemic, they allowed a safe means for interacting

FEAR RELIEVING STRATEGY #5: TECHNOLOGY AND THE RELATIONSHIP

with people. But they also provide challenges to creating a connection and a relationship. All the strategies we have discussed so far also apply to the televisit. Be sure to stop and build a connection before jumping right into business. Find out one thing about the person. Smile, make eye contact and connect. During the conversation, do not let technology distract you. Treat that person as you would if they were directly across the room from you without a computer in the middle.

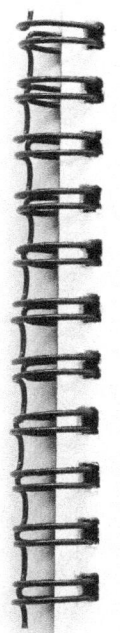

Action Steps

» *Stop what you are doing and look at the phone before answering. It helps you focus.*

» *SMILE when answering the phone. It changes your voice and sounds warm and inviting.*

» *Find a way to make a connection with the person on the other end of the line.*

» *Once you learn the name of the person on the phone, use it as much as you can to personalize the encounter.*

» *Ask people if you may put them on hold, wait for a reply and then acknowledge their patience when you return.*

» *With a televisit, remember to still build a connection with eye contact, smile, and finding out one thing about them that has nothing to do with why they called you.*

Fear Relieving Strategy #6:

Considering Different Generations have Different Expectations

When thinking about "keep me informed, keep me safe and keep me comfortable," I realized that the definition for those concepts is not the same for everyone. For those of you who have been in healthcare for a while, do you think the expectations of your patients have changed over the years of your career? When I ask this question, people usually reply that patients have many more expectations today than in the past. Perhaps you are thinking that people come in having already looked up their symptoms and know what they need. Perhaps you are thinking that they expect everything to happen fast. Perhaps you are thinking that expectations for customer service have increased. You are right. Here is a glimpse as to why I believe that is true.

I realize that there are a lot of things that make us who we are, not just when we are born. However, I also believe that there are things that happened in different generations that shaped that generation. Please know as I talk about different generations, I do not mean to stereotype but rather to learn.

Many years ago, I was rounding on an Emergency Department (ED) nursing director. She said to me, "We make all our older patients happy." When I returned to my office after our conversation, I was curious as to whether she was correct. I looked at her patient experience data sorted by age. She was exactly right. The Silent Generation was extremely happy, Baby Boomers a bit less; Generation X and Generation Y were rarely satisfied. I looked at my other adult EDs and found the exact same thing.

I went to the literature to see what was written about different generations and their expectations and saw that not much was published about patients. As I thought about what I had been teaching our leaders about our associates of different generations and their expectations, I realized our patients were not that different. Different generations have different expectations for information and for what creates a sense of caring and safety.

The Silent Generation or Radio Generation, born 1930 – 1945, experienced World War II and the Great Depression. They came back, rebuilt the country and made it strong. They conquered diseases and landed a man on the moon. They are often referred to as the Greatest Generation. This generation values hard work, respects authority and loyalty. In the workplace, this generation looks up to people with higher titles because they have earned their status. They are willing to work hard, follow directions, and stay with one organization until they retire.

As patients, this generation brings those same values into the healthcare setting. They have great respect for clinicians and their authority. They are impressed with the titles after your names. They are prepared to be loyal to you and stay with you until you retire. They listen to what you tell them and follow directions. What they want most from their provider is time. When we started implementing fast tracks in the emergency departments, this generation wrote on their

FEAR RELIEVING STRATEGY #6: CONSIDERING DIFFERENT GENERATIONS HAVE DIFFERENT EXPECTATIONS

survey, "They rushed me out." We had to change our words to say, "I know you are not feeling well and want to get you home to rest as quickly as possible."

My mother-in-law of this generation had bladder cancer. She did well with her surgery and chemotherapy. What she could not handle was getting her port accessed for her chemotherapy. When I suggested asking her physician for a prescription for EMLA to apply before going in for her treatment so she could close her eyes and not know that her port was being accessed, she replied, "If my doctor thought I needed EMLA, he would have given me EMLA." It took great convincing on my part to get her to make the call. That was the Silent Generation.

The healthcare system we work in today was created for the Silent Generation. It was totally "clinician centered," and this generation was fine with that. They would willingly sit in our waiting rooms and wait for us. Only in healthcare do waiting rooms even exist. Everyone else has lobbies and reception areas. In healthcare, we have waiting rooms, the place where you can wait until we are ready. Consider patient gowns that did not fit anyone. Why was that? Those gowns were for our ease in caring for patients.

The Baby Boomer Generation (1946-1964) was the rock the boat generation. Everything the Silent Generation valued; Baby Boomers rocked the boat. Think of what happened during this generation: Civil Rights, Women's Liberation, Vietnam, birth control. This was the generation where women entered the workforce in greater numbers. In the workplace, this generation created shared decision making–the thought that you, the leader, would make better decisions if you involved everyone.

In healthcare, they bring these same values. Shared decision making is important. My physician sent me a text once suggesting I start on a statin. My immediate response was, "Can we talk about it?" I laughed and reflected on my mother-in-law who would not ask for EMLA, and here I am challenging my physician on a statin.

Baby Boomers are also the forever young generation. Think of all the industries that have been created to keep this generation feeling young and healthy forever. Many years ago, I injured my back and my physical therapist asked me about my goals for therapy. My response was, "I want the pain to go away so I can go back to Yoga and Zumba and my life." I wanted to be returned to my same state of health as before my injury. Thanks to my physical therapist, I accomplished my goal, but I think about baby boomers who have a heart attack or stroke and want to return to their previous state. They may become easily frustrated if they do not.

Baby Boomers were the first generation to view themselves as consumers of healthcare. The Silent Generation was loyal to their family doctor, but Baby Boomers realized if they did not like their doctor, they could find another one.

Most of all, it is important to remember that the generations are more alike than different. Everyone has fears and wants the same 3 things: Keep me informed, keep me safe, and keep me comfortable.

Gen X (1965-1979) was the next generation and the children of the Baby Boomers. For many of this generation, both parents worked outside the home. They came home to an empty house at the end of the school day. They did their homework, made themselves a snack and grew up to be an independent generation. In the workplace, this generation is not impressed with rank and credentials, rather competence. They do not care to get together as a team and solve problems; they prefer to work independently. In healthcare, those same values are apparent. They are not impressed with merely the clinician's credentials but rather their competence. When we share information with this generation, then they know that we know what we are doing. They are looking to us for knowledge so that they can identify the right plan of care for themselves. And this is the shift from "tell me what to do" (Silent Generation) to "let's talk about it" (Baby Boomers) to "educate me so I make the right decisions" (Gen X).

Gen Y (1980-1994) has had technology at their fingertips since they were quite small. Technology provides information and speed. This

FEAR RELIEVING STRATEGY #6: CONSIDERING DIFFERENT GENERATIONS HAVE DIFFERENT EXPECTATIONS

generation is often thought of as "Gen WHY" because they always want to know and strive to know the why. Our challenges with this generation are to find ways to provide them with good information. They like being connected and would go to their healthcare system website for information if it was readily available. The need for speed is another opportunity for healthcare since we do not move at the same speed as this generation is used to. It is important to set realistic expectations, so they do not feel frustrated or forgotten.

Lastly, I often reflect on the stack of paper we provide at discharge. This is a generation that does not relate to paper. They look at us as environmentally insensitive for killing a tree to provide simple instructions about home care. With anything important, this generation is likely to take a picture of it with their phone and throw the paper away. We need to figure out ways to get this information to them electronically.

Gen Z (1995-2009) data is just emerging about their expectations with healthcare. It appears that a growing number prefer digital encounters. Technology will be crucial for meeting their needs. They want flexibility, transparency and convenience. How does our current healthcare system meet the needs of this generation during scary and stressful times?

As you think about each generation, I hope you understand the growing importance and significance of information and control. My reflection on this topic is that is why patient and family-centered care is so important and yet so challenging for us. We are used to a healthcare system that revolves around the providers. With each generation, there is a desire for more and more control over their health and information. I believe that is why handoffs at the bedside and frequently rounding on patients are so important to them. With more control and information, the generations that follow the Silent Generation feel safer and more comfortable.

Action Steps

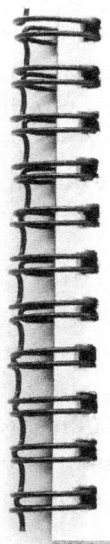

» Always strive to be patient and family centered. A healthcare system that is provider centered is no longer viable.

» Recognize each generation following the Silent Generation wants increasingly more control and information.

» Learn how to adapt our processes to meet the needs of different generations.

Part 2

Healthcare Team Members are People Too!

We tend to focus on the needs and fears of patients and families. Sometimes we forget that our healthcare team members are also people with fears, concerns and anxiety. When the healthcare team members are afraid, it can impact the work they do.

In the Spring of 2020 at the beginning of the COVID-19 pandemic, one of my favorite nurses, Rachel, told me that she was worried. She was worried she would make a mistake because she could not concentrate or stay focused. She was having trouble thinking clearly. I instantly realized she had a snake on her head. If patients and families cannot hear information, concentrate, or focus when they are scared, why would our clinicians during a pandemic be any different? Rachel was scared. She had a snake her head, and it was impacting her.

When I mentioned the snake, she confirmed that she was indeed scared. She was afraid of getting sick, afraid of bringing the virus home to her family. Worried she was not taking all the right precautions. Worried about keeping her patients safe. Challenged with how to keep families who were not allowed in the hospital informed about their loved one.

Just like our patients and families, I believe our clinicians and staff are worried, anxious and fearful. They also want those same three things as our patients and families: Keep me informed. Keep me safe. Keep me comfortable.

With the onset of COVID-19, information changed by the moment as we were learning how to deal with the pandemic. Strategies for patient care kept evolving. Precautions to keep staff safe also continue to evolve. The fear patients and families were experiencing caused anger and that added increased stress to the team. They needed information continuously. They needed reassurance and support from their leaders to feel safe and comfortable at work.

At times of great change and great uncertainty, it is more important than ever for leaders to round on their team, both informally in a group and one on one. How are they doing? What are their biggest concerns and worries? What can you as leader do to help them? What ideas do they have to improve the situation?

Many hospital presidents sent out daily updates to their teams about what was happening in the hospital and their concerns. They sent out positive stories that would keep the team motivated. These updates did not need to be fancy but frequent, as transparency alleviates fear. Just like our patients and families need frequent information and updates on how they are doing to decrease their anxiety, so do clinicians and the healthcare team.

In my over 40 years as a nurse, 2020 was my first pandemic. However, there are lots of other times when I experienced that fear.

Other Scary Times

New Job

Think back to the first day of a new job. How were you feeling? I would imagine a great deal of excitement and perhaps a bit of anxiety. What were your fears? What were the most important things your new leader or new team could do for you to alleviate your fears? Perhaps you are thinking, "keep me informed, keep me safe, keep me comfortable."

Every time I have started a new position, I worried about whether I was competent enough for the new job. I wondered how they did things. I wondered if people would like me, be nice to me and include me on the team.

Keep me informed: I think it is important for organizations to carefully plan the orientation to the department. New employee orientation always occurs in organizations and covers major policies, human resources onboarding and other important global information. But what happens in the department? Do we give the new person a mentor, a buddy to make sure they know how things are done, where things are located, who to go to for help? Do we show people how to request their schedule preferences and such mundane things as where and when to eat lunch? Do we introduce them to other team members? Do we share those unwritten secrets that we know make the job easier?

Feeling safe: Just as we do not know our patients' fears since they are different for each patient, a new team member has their unique fears as well. It is important to ask them what they need. When I was a new nurse, I was terrified of having to place a needle into a child, either for an injection, to draw blood or to start an IV. My preceptor asked me what was my greatest worry that I needed help with, and I told her. She immediately found as many opportunities as possible for me to draw blood, start IVs, or give injections. Her goal was to get that snake off my head so that I could focus on all the other things she needed to teach me.

As a result, I not only became proficient with needle sticks on children, I became a Pediatric Hematology/Oncology nurse where that was a large part of my job. I learned that skill mixed with compassion and empathy would help a child cope with the procedure. I needed to address my fear so that I would be able to focus on the children's fears. If you have the privilege of mentoring someone who is new to their role or to their position, find out what is the most important thing you can do to minimize their greatest worries or concerns.

Feeling comfortable: getting to know people. When my son, who is now a physician, was an 18-year-old high school graduate waiting to start college, he got a job in a hospital as an anesthesia tech for the summer. The tech who was orienting him could have introduced him to the surgeons and anesthesiologists as an 18-year-old going off to college, but instead chose to introduce him as the new anesthesia tech on the team who will be a doctor one day. The anesthesiologists took him under their wing and taught him things I am sure he would not have learned if he was just "a kid going off to college in the fall."

He returned during every school break and the physicians in the operating room checked on his progress toward medical school. This

OTHER SCARY TIMES

was an invaluable opportunity, all because of the way he was introduced at the onset. How does your department introduce new team members?

What if someone reached out before your first day to welcome you? What if the team sent a card to your home before the first day? What if there was a banner in the department welcoming you when you arrived? When our daughter was 4, we moved to San Antonio in late September. She was starting a new preschool, having left all her friends on the east coast. We arrived in San Antonio a day earlier than expected and went to the preschool to show it to her. When we arrived at her classroom, there on the floor was a star with her name on it in the circle, just like each of the other students. They had been anxiously awaiting the arrival of the new student. Imagine how welcomed and comfortable our daughter felt. First impressions matter to team members and clinicians. Try to imagine what their first few moments are like?

How can we help new team members feel informed, safe, and comfortable in their new position?

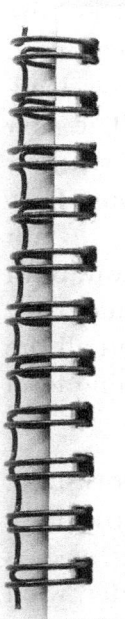

Action Steps

» *Help them become part of the team. Do not just orient them to the organization.*

» *Provide new team members with a mentor to help them feel safe, informed and comfortable.*

» *Find out what are they most worried about and address that concern as soon as possible.*

» *Find out something about them that has nothing to do with their job.*

» *Introduce them to patients, families, and team members in a way that makes them feel safe and comfortable.*

» *Find a creative way to welcome new team members to your department.*

New Leaders

Can you remember the last time you got a new leader? A new boss? One of the things I have learned from working with teams is just how stressful it is when a leader leaves the organization or team. Whether the team liked the previous leader or was happy to see that leader leave, it does not matter. The uncertainty of the leader leaving and a new one joining the team leads to stress and worry. The team wonders, who is that new leader? What do they expect from us? What are they going to change? What is their leadership style? What are their hot buttons that I should never push? While the team members are worrying about all these things, it impacts their effectiveness.

It is important for the leader to get to know each person on the team as an individual, to learn something about them that has nothing to do with their job. Learn about their family, their priorities, their career goals, their hobbies, how they like to be recognized and how they prefer to communicate.

> *Every great dream begins with a dreamer. Always remember, you have within you the strength, the patience, and the passion to reach for the stars to change the world.*
>
> Harriet Tubman

A jumpstart or transition workshop is a great tool for helping the team and the new leader get to the know each other. The team learns about the new leader's vision and expectations. The new leader can quickly get to know their new team and their expectations. They can learn what gives the team a source of pride, what they do not want to change and what obstacles and barriers get in their way. Both the team and the leader can learn so much in a few hours, build trust and a relationship, create a shared vision for the future; and all the things that help get the team back to their highest functioning level as quickly as possible.

There are many ways to achieve success with this type of workshop. It is often facilitated by an objective, skilled facilitator. It provides a means for the team to share with the leader what is working, what is not working, what they need and want from their new leader, what

OTHER SCARY TIMES

questions and fears they have, and what they foresee happening in the next few months that the leader might want to know. The second half of the session allows the leader to share their leadership credo, their operating style, their core beliefs, their vision for the department and their communication style. Having these conversations puts the team at ease and gets the snake off their head so they can be their best.

I was facilitating a transition workshop for a team one day when they mentioned to the new leader that they were frustrated that the 3-hole punch had been broken for many months. That new leader stopped at an office supply store on her way home that day and bought a new 3-hole punch. Imagine how the team felt the very next day to have one of their biggest frustrations immediately fixed. Imagine how that eased their worries about their new leader.

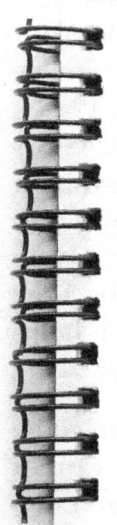

Action Steps

» *Get to know each team member as a person, not only as a professional.*
» *Plan a transition workshop for the team.*
» *Share your vision with the team.*

Change

Most people do not immediately love and embrace change. Change in healthcare is happening at a fast pace today. As leaders, how do you help your team through change? Resistance to change is often rooted in fear. For example, as a nurse, I know that getting a new catheter for starting IVs can be so stressful. Nurses have actually stashed old catheters so they could go back to them after the new ones appeared. Many people shudder when they learn that their documentation system is changing. Why? Perhaps they are afraid that they will not be competent with the new process or equipment. Perhaps it is the fear that it will take longer. Perhaps they do not understand why they need to change.

Consider the three things people want when they are afraid and apply them to the change process: Keep me informed. Keep me safe. Keep me comfortable.

The sooner you can engage the team in understanding the WHY for the change and allowing them to participate in the HOW we make the change, the more successful I believe we will be as leaders. I often say that I do not like change unless it is my idea. Remember my story as a new nurse going to the chief nurse with all the changes I thought would help the children? The people who are doing the job know how to best implement change and feel valued, comfortable and safe when their ideas are heard. As they become engaged in the implementation, it helps diminish the fear of the unknown.

Do not go where the path may lead; go instead where there is no path and leave a trail.

Ralph Waldo Emerson

Information shared during the change process is critical. As a leader, you cannot overcommunicate. Remember that communication goes both ways. I believe it is important to communicate not just before the change, but during and after as well. Make sure everyone is confident that they have the knowledge, tools and vision to successfully create the desired results. Share information as you get it and listen

OTHER SCARY TIMES

to all concerns and ideas. Show the team the results of the change and how the effort made a difference.

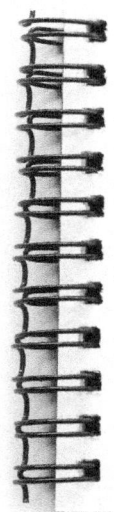

Action Steps

» Keep the team informed: communicate, communicate, communicate.

» Always share the WHY about the change and involve the team in the HOW whenever possible.

» Share results that demonstrate HOW the change made a difference.

Words Matter:
Their Impact on the Team

Remember my Southwest Airlines story that words matter? They matter to us and to our team as well as to our patients. How often do we come to work saying, "This is going to be a Monday! Look at the patient load. This is going to be a bad day.'" What if we change the words we say to ourselves? "I am going to make a difference today! I am going to find three things to be grateful for today." At the end of each day as you are driving home, do you berate yourself all the way home with all the things you did not do well or could have done better? Instead, I encourage you to ask yourself, "How did I make a difference today? Who did I make a difference for?" The work you do is so important. Every day you make a difference for someone. Focus on the things that will help you feel fulfilled and stop your negative self-talk that will only add to your compassion fatigue. When you set an intention to make a difference that day or if you know at the end of the day you need to find three things you are grateful for, it's amazing how your brain begins to focus on those things.

One day I was driving in heavy traffic and running late. Of course, we are never stuck in heavy traffic when we have extra time. I found

THERE'S A SNAKE ON MY HEAD!

I was gripping the steering wheel tightly and my shoulders were up around my ears. Suddenly, I realized that it did not matter how tightly I gripped the wheel, I would still be just as late. So, I took a deep breath, relaxed my grip on the wheel, turned up the radio and sang at the top of my lungs. When I arrived, I was still late, but I was not ready to bite the head off the first person I saw. I had not changed the situation; I had merely changed my attitude. We often do not have control over what happens to us over the day, but we have control over our attitude. At some point, the day will end, and you will get to go home. How do you cope with what happens in the meantime?

I believe the attitude you choose will impact how you see things and the energy you have to cope with whatever comes your way. I have learned that my attitude affects the others around me. Have you ever arrived at work feeling positive and happy, excited about the day ahead and then greeted by someone who did not share your outlook? The negative energy experienced from that other person can impact your positivity. I do not want to impact others in a negative manner, so I strive to choose a positive attitude. I also believe it can impact our patients. They surely do not need a negative attitude from their care team. They already have their own problems which are usually significantly worse than anything I am experiencing.

Change your thoughts and you change your world.

Norman Vincent Peale

Now, what about the words we say to our team at work? When someone tells you that the patient in Room 10 is difficult, don't you walk into the room already prepared for them to be difficult, even before you say hello? Once that thought is in your head, your brain works hard to prove you right.

Choose your words wisely in huddle. If someone declares, "this is going to be a bad day," it impacts the whole team. Everyone's brain hears the message and looks for ways the day is bad. If we tell the team, this will be a great day or maybe busy today, but we are a great team and we can do this, it changes the view of the day. And do not forget to share words of gratitude in huddle at the end of a busy day.

WORDS MATTER: THEIR IMPACT ON THE TEAM

This sends your team home knowing the work they do is important and makes a difference.

I will never forget being in a huddle one morning at change of shift. The shift was busy with only one certified nursing assistant (CNA) on duty for the whole unit. Her head was resting on the top of the counter during the meeting. At the conclusion of the huddle, the charge nurse said, "Before we leave, I want to thank our CNA. She was the only CNA on all night and never stopped running. I do not know what we would have done without you tonight. You are our hero!" The CNA lifted her head off the counter and smiled. I just knew if the charge nurse had not shared those kind words, she would have gone home that night thinking she had failed. She had failed her patients and her team. I am sure she was unable to provide the level of care she had hoped to provide. She may have even started thinking about whether this was the job for her or whether she wanted to come back again this next night. Instead, she was the hero. The team would be lost without her.

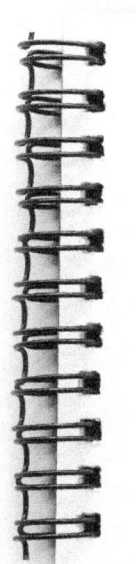

Action Steps

» *Find three things to be grateful for each day.*

» *Choose a positive attitude. It impacts your team, your patients and yourself.*

» *Show gratitude to your team. Let them know you appreciate them.*

» *Watch the words you say to yourself and others. Your brain and their brain are listening.*

Final Thoughts

I have a few special stories to leave you with in the appendix. Before I do, let me close with one of my favorite quotes. It is from Mr. Fred Rogers. He said,

"If you could only sense how important you are to the lives of those you meet; how important you can be to the people you may never even dream of. There is something of yourself that you leave at every meeting with another person."

I think this is true in healthcare. As a leader, a team member, and a clinician, we impact the lives of those we meet every day. How can we help people feel safe with us and feel cared about? That is our challenge. Most of us have had the opportunity to walk into a restaurant or store and have someone come up to us and say with great excitement, "Do you remember me? You took care of me." We usually smile and nod and say, "Of course, how are you?" even if we do not remember them. We may forget them, but they will never forget us. As a leader you impact the lives of your team members and the lives of their families as well. You never know when you are inspiring someone to grow and learn. I have had the privilege and honor of having people come back to me many years later and share the influence I have had on their life or their career. It is surprising and quite humbling.

THERE'S A SNAKE ON MY HEAD!

During my first year of nursing, I remember driving to work thinking how lucky I was to be paid for doing what I was so passionate about. Almost 45 years later, I never forgot the privilege of working with patients and families and team members at the most vulnerable and important moments in their lives. People never forget the people who have cared for them. It is an honor and a privilege.

Every day focus on your purpose.
Remember WHY you do what you do.
We don't get burned out because of WHAT we do.
We get burned out because we forget WHY we do it.

Jon Gordon

Postscript:
Another Snake

As I completed the draft of the book, I felt joy and relief for having all my thoughts on paper. THEN…it hit me. I got stuck. I did not know what to do next. I wondered how do you get a book edited and published? Would anyone want to read it? Is there enough information in the book?

Fortunately, my husband Barry and dear friend, Joe Tye, would not let it rest. One day as I explained to Joe why the book was never going to be printed, he looked at me and said, "I can see that snake on your head." WOW! What powerful words and so true.

Try to be a rainbow in someone else's cloud.

Maya Angelou

At that point, Joe connected me with Lisa Peterson, a very kind, patient and knowledgeable person who assured me she would walk with me through the whole process of design, editing and printing. What did I need when I had that snake on my head? I needed information. I needed to feel safe and comfortable. Lisa did just that for me. Watch out for those snakes in your lives that can paralyze and stop you in your tracks! Be there to help and encourage others when you see that snake on their head.

Stories and Experiences

I had two people share stories with me of experiences they had with clinicians that made a difference for them during extremely scary times. I would like to share these stories with you.

A Modern Day Florence
By Joe Tye

Late in 2015, I traveled to a rural Texas hospital for what was to have been a 3-day series of events. I'd been feeling terrible but wasn't about to stand up a client. When I arrived to meet the executive team the evening before we were to start, the chief nursing officer took one look at me and said he was taking me to the emergency room, not to the board room. After a CT scan, I was diagnosed with acute diverticulitis and admitted. They took great care of me. One of the hospital housekeepers even went to the local Walmart and bought me a pair of sweatpants. But after three days, against the better judgement of my physician, I checked out because I had a plane ticket and commitments back home.

Several hours after arriving home, I was in the Emergency Department at the University of Iowa Hospitals and Clinics. From there I was admitted to an inpatient unit where I stayed for the next nine days. Midway through my stay, the senior surgery resident came into my room and told me that since the medical treatment hadn't been working, they wanted to do surgery. She said that they would excise part of my colon and put me on a colostomy bag. If all went well, she told me, I would only need to wear the colostomy bag for a year or so. If things did not go well, she continued, the colostomy bag would be with me for the rest of my life. No way, I exclaimed. I would rather die. That, she replied with a straight face, would be another option.

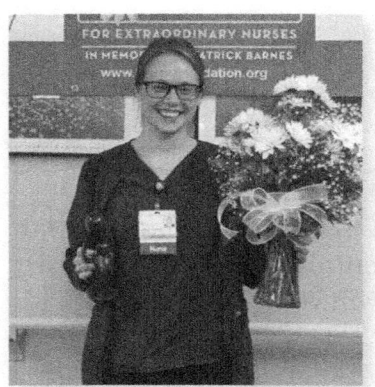

Needless to say, this was deeply depressing. Several hours later, when I was at my lowest point emotionally, Shelly Lacy – a relatively new nursing school graduate who'd been my primary caregiver – came in and sat on the edge of my bed. For the next half hour, she reassured me that this would not be the end of life as I'd known it. She also explained what the risks might be should I elect against having the surgery. By the time she left my room, I was in a much more positive frame of mind. Five days later, I walked out of the hospital with my colon intact. It is still intact.

While the physicians did a good job of explaining the medical carpentry of the surgery, it was Shelly who explained at a practical level how it would work, described how I could manage the inconvenience and continue to do my work. She shared examples of other people who had accommodated themselves to a colostomy. She convinced me that whether I had the surgery, it was my choice to make. That contribution was, I believe, more important to my healing than the medical treatment. I nominated Shelly for a DAISY Award, which she won. The day I attended her award ceremony, the thought struck me that from somewhere Florence Nightingale was looking on with a proud smile.

POSTSCRIPT: STORIES AND EXPERIENCES

Alex and Her Dad, Alejandra Mascorro

A dear colleague of mine, Alex, shared this story with me.

Her dad, her best friend, was visiting her from out of town in 2013, when he came down with a quick and sudden illness. On a Sunday, he came into the ER scared, confused, and alone, with his wife driving in from 250 miles away. The ER nurse explained everything to Alex and him, acknowledging their fear. Both the doctor and the nurse were excellent.

Due to the grave nature of the situation, her dad was quickly admitted to the ICU, still very confused and at times, had to be restrained. The staff joked with him, calling him their "BFF." They prayed with him and treated him like family. The ICU team recognized his fears and his wife's. They constantly explained everything they were doing in very simple terms. They sat at his bedside and connected with the family. They comforted everyone. Alex says, "I will never forget them."

Four days after staying by his side for 24 hours around the clock, Alex and her family were exhausted. They asked the night nurse to please watch over him as they all decided to leave him for the night. That night nurse was trusted by the family. They felt safe enough to leave him and go home to sleep. When the family returned, the nurse told the family, "I stayed with him all night. I held his hand all shift. I could relate to him, as my father had a heart attack, and someone stayed with him. Someone did it for my dad, so I did it for yours."

Five days after admission, her father, her best friend, took his last breath at 3:03 pm.

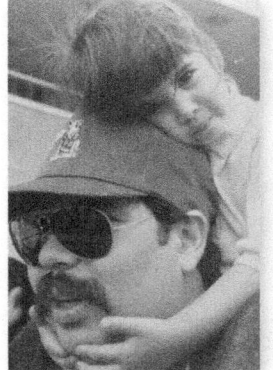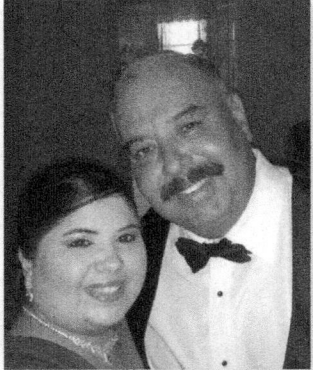

Little Alex and then one month before her father died.

THERE'S A SNAKE ON MY HEAD!

Alex is a clinician at that same hospital.

I asked her what keeps her there. She merely replied, "I came back because someone did that for my dad, so I will do it for someone else's."

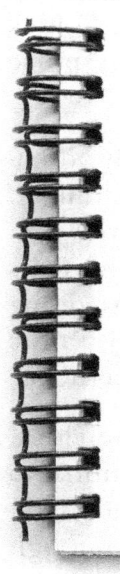

Remember

» Every patient you are privileged to care for is someone's cell phone person. The work you do is so important.
» Every day you make a difference and touch people's lives.
» Never lose your "WHY"!

References

Fear

1. "Fears of Parents When Their Child Is a Patient" https://www.theberylinstitute.org/store/viewproduct.aspx?ID=15744255
2. "Communication strategies to mitigate fear and suffering among COVID-19 patients isolated in the ICU and their families" https://www.ncbi.nlm.nih.gov/pmc/articles/PMC7196381
3. "Patients' fear of physicians and perceptions of physicians' cultural competence in healthcare" https://www.tandfonline.com/doi/full/10.1080/17538068.2017.1287389?scroll=top&needAccess=true
4. Webster, Anna. (2011) "Easing Patient Fears Can Raise HCAHPS Scores" Health Leaders Media.
5. Maslow, A. H. A. (1943) "Theory of Human Motivation" Psychological Review, 50, 370- 396.
6. Steimer, Thierry. (2002) "The Biology of fear- and anxiety-related behaviors" Dialogues in Clinical Neurosciences, 4(3) 231- 249.
7. Kornusky, Jennifer. (2016) "Communicating with a Patient Who is Fearful" CINAHL Nursing Guide. Ebsco.com.
8. Mylod, Deirdre; and Lee, Thomas. (2013) "A Framework for Reducing Suffering in Healthcare" Harvard Business Review.
9. McLeod, Jane and Tetzloff, Sue. (2015) "Value of Purposeful Rounding" American Nurse Today.
10. Gregory, S., Tan, D., Tilrico M., Edwardson, N., Gamm, L. (2014) "Bedside Shift Repot: What does the Evidence Say?" Journal of Nursing Administration.

11. McAllen, E., Stephens, K., Swanson-Biearman, B., Kerr, K., Whiteman, K. (2018) "Moving Shift Report to the Bedside" Online Journal of Issues in Nursing.

12. Moore, Walter; Buckley, Peter; Engels, Nettie; O'Meara, Christine; Sodomka, Patricia; Roberson, Bernard. (February 2010) "Navigating Patient and Family Centered Rounds: A Guide to Achieving Success" Institute for Patient and Family Centered Care website (IPFCC.org)

13. Colleen Sweeney Resources: sweeneyhealthcareenterprises.com
"160 Ways to Empathize"
"Dear Caregivers: Thoughts from an Everyday Patient" (video or poster)
"The Exam: Getting Inside a Patient's Head" (video)

Patient Experience and Associate Experience

Dempsey, Christina. (2018) *Antidote to Suffering*

Spiegelman, Paul and Berrett, Britt. (2013) *Patients Come Second. Leading Change by Changing the Way You Lead*

Studer, Quint. (2003) *Hardwiring Excellence*

Freiberg, Kevin and Jackie. (1997) *Nuts! Southwest Airlines' Crazy Recipe for Business and Personal Success*

Communication

Chou, C. and Cooley, L. (2018) *Communication Rx. Transforming Healthcare Through Relationship Centered Communication*

Covey, Stephen R. (1989) *The 7 Habits of Highly Effective People: Powerful Lessons in Personal Change.*

Positivity

Achor, Shawn. (2010) *The Happiness Advantage*

Tye, Joe. (2009, 2014, 2017, 2020) *The Florence Prescription*

REFERENCES

Generations

Lancaster, L. and Stillman, D. (2005) *When Generations Collide*

Gravett, L. and Throckmorton, R. (2007) *Bridging the Generation Gap*

About the Author

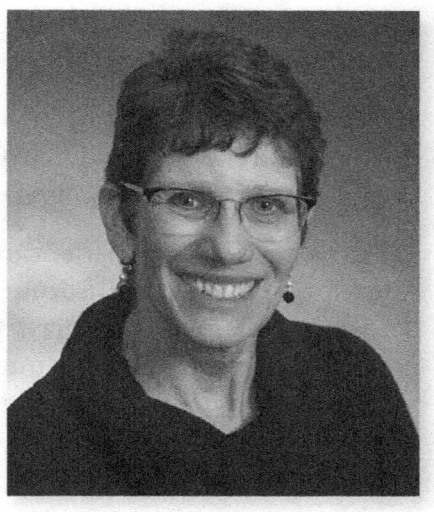

Mindy Spigel's passion is helping people create meaningful connections as a leader, a team member, while caring for customers. She enjoys helping leaders build strong teams and exceptional work environments.

She is committed to helping teams communicate, respect each other, and work together effectively. It is her desire to alleviate fears, build trust, and create an extraordinary experience for all.

Mindy Spigel is proud to be a nurse with experience working in both inpatient and outpatient settings. As an educator, Mindy has taught in both academic and clinical settings. Mindy has served on the faculty of two universities: University of Alabama in Birmingham with a joint appointment to the School of Nursing and the School of Medicine and at Christopher Newport College where she served as the pediatric faculty member at the College of Nursing. Mindy was also the Director of Education for a hospital where she was responsible for staff, patient and communication education.

Mindy has been honored to have presented at numerous national, state and local conferences and provided consultation and coaching to various organizations.

Mindy worked at CHRISTUS Santa Rosa and The Children's Hospital of San Antonio for almost 29 years as the Director of Organizational Effectiveness and the Director of Patient Experience. In these roles Mindy facilitated leadership development workshops and provided individual coaching to the leadership team. She loves facilitating transition workshops as leaders onboard, as well as facilitating team building and team interventions to create an exceptional work environment. She loves coaching physicians, leaders and other clinicians in creating an exceptional patient and family experience. Mindy has been recognized as a Certified Patient Experienced Professional (CPXP).

Mindy has recently completed and published a research study on the "Fears of Parents When Their Child is a Patient" with support from the Beryl Institute. *There's a Snake on My Head!* is her first book.

Mindy is active in the patient experience community. Currently, she is serving on the Beryl Institute Patient Experience Policy Forum for Patient and Family Centered Care, Academy for Communication in Healthcare Research Committee and University of Houston in San Antonio, C. T. Bauer College of Business Customer Experience Advisory Panel.

Thank You!

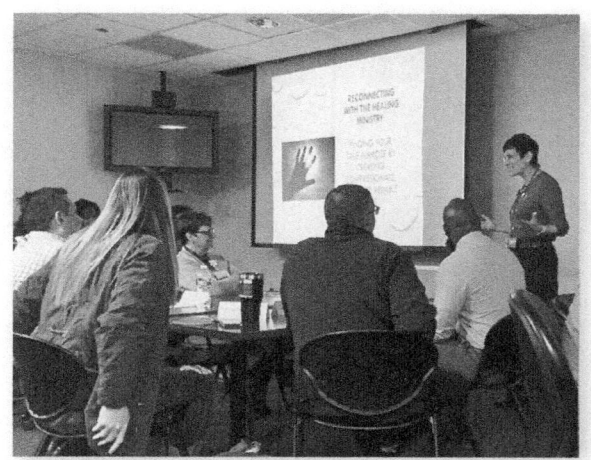

Thank you so much for reading my first book! I hope you found it to be insightful and helpful in assisting you with looking at the patient and family experience in a new light. I hope the next time you encounter a "difficult patient" you will be able to see that they are scared and find a way to help them feel safe. Remembering too, that there are times when the healthcare team may be afraid and also needs steps taken to put them at ease.

It was a joy to share my research, teachings, and learnings with you. If you found this book to be helpful, please encourage your friends and colleagues to read it.

I would also love it if you would go to Amazon and leave a review. Your feedback helps us reach more people and makes a difference to those who are considering reading the book and learning about ways to help their patients and families.

Again, thank you for sharing my journey with me and thank you for what you do every day.

Mindy

What's Next?

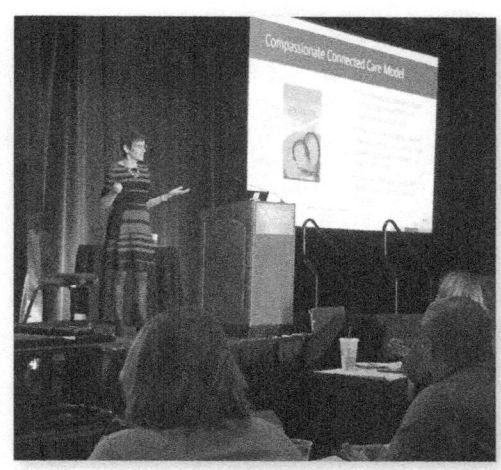

If you found this book to be helpful for your practice, you may be wondering, what else? I invite you to reach out to me. I would love to help you and your team create a safe and comfortable experience for patients, families and the healthcare team. Some of my favorite speaking engagements include the following topics:

- There's Snake on My Head
- Engaging, Motivating and Retaining your Team
- Managing Through Change
- Managing Difficult Conversations
- Effectively Managing Customer Complaints
- Taking Care of Yourself
- Building Strong Teams

Please reach out to me through **MindySpigel.com** and schedule a call so we can talk about your specific needs and how to apply these strategies in your organization.

Download Your Gift

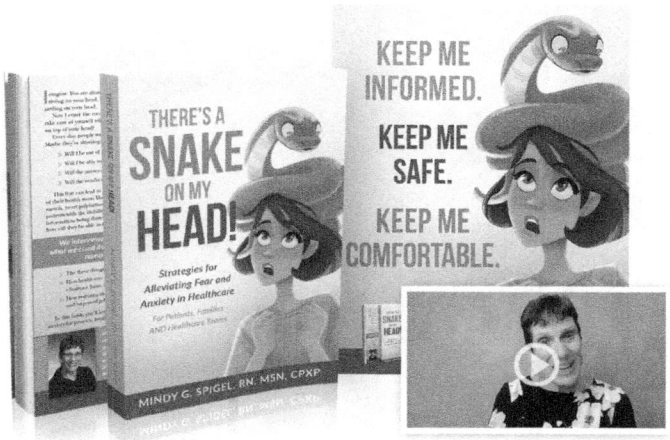

As a thank you for reading my book, I'd like to give you access to the companion training video and poster for *There's a Snake on My Head!*

In the video you'll learn:

- » Simple techniques to help put patients and families at ease without adding time to your day.
- » How they could feel more satisfied with the care they are already receiving.
- » Why they cannot hear what we are telling them, which may affect their compliance.
- » What can impact the effectiveness and job satisfaction of the healthcare team and how to resolve it.

Use the poster as a gentle reminder of what patients, families and healthcare teams need on a daily basis.

Visit **MindySpigel.com/gift**

Made in the USA
Monee, IL
17 November 2023

46824373R00057